The Wireless

We would certainly all agree that health and environmental ~~~~
has been increasing over the past two decades. Organic foods, yoga
centers, mind body programs, health clubs and the healing arts have
proliferated. Even healthy 'fast food' restaurants have arrived, and
large food brands are beginning to go GMO-free. As consumers, we
are increasingly making 'green' choices that support mother Earth, and
which respect our intrinsic relationship with it.

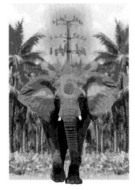

Why then, despite all this interest in health and
in living 'green', do we have over 133 million
people with a chronic illness in the U.S.—
approximately 45% of the population[1], and
growing? Promotion of 'prevention,' and, more
recently, 'rationing' care, has been the response
to high costs driven by chronic illnesses. But
in looking for solutions to costs, we may be
'missing the forest for the trees', and also not
understanding the true meaning of prevention.

Prevention

The word 'prevention' rings hollow *unless one is seeking to eliminate
the factors that can lead to disease in the first place*. These include
unhealthy lifestyle choices, how we respond to stress, heavy metal
and chemical toxicity, exposures to electromagnetic fields (EMFs),
petroleum-based fertilizers, the weed killer glyphosate, GMO
foods, poor nutrition, difficult relationships, etc. Today, 'prevention'
instead typically means early detection of disease with tests like
mammography, pap smear and PSA; manipulation of one's physiology
with pharmaceuticals and vaccines (which can have their own negative
side effects); and, perhaps, depending on the doctor, advice to eat more
vegetables and exercise. *But prevention in the full sense of the word
means something else entirely, and we ignore this at our peril.*

**True prevention means first removing from our lives those things
that create biological dis-regulation and dis-ease, while identifying
and proactively increasing the things that create balance and wellness.**

The word 'prevention' rings hollow unless one is seeking to eliminate the factors that can lead to disease in the first place.

The Unseen Elephant

A health care system that does not advocate for dramatic reduction in cell phone and wireless radiation exposures ignores over six decades of scientific research showing biological and health effects from electromagnetic fields, including recent research from the NIH.[2][3] It ignores repeated resolutions from scientists and physicians worldwide calling for caution, and the classification of cell phone and wireless radiation (radiofrequency radiation or RFR) by the WHO's International Agency for Research on Cancer (IARC) as a 'Possible Carcinogen' (Group 2B)[4]. It ignores the experience of people in every corner of the globe with life-altering, sometimes debilitating, symptoms from acute and chronic exposures to wireless technologies. And, it turns a blind eye to the DNA-damage consequences of these wireless conveniences for ourselves today, as well as for future generations.

In parallel with the growth of chronic illnesses since the 1990s, it is hard not to notice that the amount of wireless communication infrastructure in our midst has been exploding. Four and a half billion people use a cell phone today, whereas in the early 1990s most people didn't own a cell phone. There are now millions of cell towers radiating the planet, many hundreds of millions WiFi networks[5] and billions of wireless devices connected to them.[6]

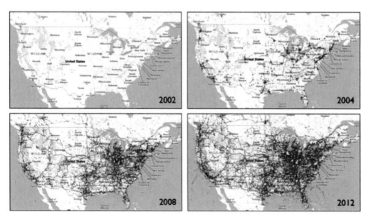

Source: Wigle.net

In parallel with the growth of chronic illnesses since the 1990s, it is hard not to notice that the amount of wireless communication infrastructure in our midst has been exploding.

Certainly, there has also been growth in other environmental pollutants during this period, and many people are over-drugged and suffer from drug interactions, with costly side effects, that also drive total costs. For example, on average, individuals 65 to 69 years old take nearly 14 prescriptions per year.[7] But, as a society, we are not fully 'seeing' the important EMF issue in the background, which has direct effects on biology and leads to a wide range of acute and chronic health issues.

In addition to the many known biological effects, EMFs also have interactive effects with man-made chemicals, heavy metals and microorganisms in our bodies, and with metal implants and amalgams, exacerbating the biological effects. And, importantly, unknown to most people, radiofrequency radiation can impact drug actions. The radiation can both enhance and decrease the efficacy of a drug, impacting the drug actions of amphetamines, anxiolytics, opiates and alcohol to name just a few.[8] Few prescribing physicians are focused on this, or asking patients who take pharmaceutical drugs about their exposures to wireless devices and infrastructure. Overprescribing pharmaceuticals to address electrosensitivity symptoms is one of the resulting travesties, and drugs will never solve the problem.

Stressing Our Biology

Our bodies are attempting to cope in an *entirely different* milieu than the one in which most adults today were raised. Biology is being continually stressed from the acute and cumulative effects of these pulsing energy fields, and responds by creating stress proteins, as with any other kind of stressor. Is it any wonder, then, that the incidence of chronic illness has accelerated since the early 1990s along side the rapid proliferation of these technologies?

Here is a graph showing six hours of radiofrequency radiation exposures to an individual in New York City wearing a portable dosimeter on March 1, 2016. The graph shows the extraordinary density of electromagnetic field exposures of different kinds, the variable nature of the pulsing and peaks, and that exposures today are way above safety guidelines based on biological scientific evidence[9] (peaking, in this particular case, in fact, way above the top of the graph).

Our bodies are attempting to cope in an entirely different milieu than the one in which most adults today were raised...Biology is being continually stressed from the acute and cumulative effects of these pulsing energy fields.

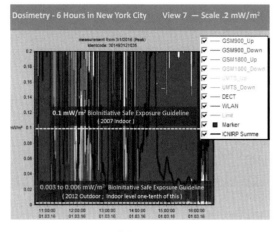

It should be noted that since the 1990s we have seen tremendous growth in neurological and psychological disorders, such as depression and bipolar disease, autoimmune diseases, inflammatory conditions, autism, ADHD, sleep disorders, chronic fatigue, diabetes and metabolic conditions. In children, we are seeing increases in psychiatric disorders, psychotropic medication use, chronic medical conditions, delinquency, addictions, aggression, sensory integration issues, and disability filings.[10] And we are seeing a growing number of reproductive issues and decreased fertility.[11]

The BioInitiative Report (much of which was later published in *Pathophysiology*) synthesizes the key findings of thousands of scientific studies showing biological effects from electromagnetic fields.[12] The U.K. publication, *Electromagnetic Sensitivity and Electromagnetic Hypersensitivity*, available through E.S.-U.K.[13] contains references to 1,800 studies showing effects of low-intensity exposures. There exists decades of military Radiofrequency (RF) research showing risk, much foreign research, and even an industry-funded review, *"Mobile Telecommunications and Health,"* prepared by the Ecolog Institute, which was issued in 2000 and lays out the known risks in great detail, including DNA risks, cancer risks and risks to children.[14]

The International Commission for Electromagnetic Safety (ICEMS) and the National Institute for the Study and Control of Cancer and Environmental Diseases 'Bernardino Ramazzini', published a report, *"Non-thermal Effects and Mechanisms of Interaction Between Electromagnetic Fields and Living Matter"* in 2010. This was an international effort by scientists to compile what was known at that time about the biological effects and mechanisms of action, and included studies showing EMFs create oxidative stress, blood-brain

"In children, we are seeing increases in psychiatric disorders, psychotropic medication use, chronic medical conditions, delinquency, addictions, aggression, sensory integration issues, and disability filings."

— **Victoria Dunckley, MD**
Child Psychiatrist & Author,
"Reset Your Child's Brain"

barrier permeability, genotoxic and fertility effects, heat shock (or stress) proteins, changes in the autonomic nervous system (ANS) and in neurotransmitters, and much more.[15]

The millions of magnetic crystals per gram of brain tissue that orient us to the Earth's magnetic field (as high as 100 million crystals per gram in brain membranes) are also affected by artificial electromagnetic fields and are believed to be playing a role, as well, in the biological dis-regulation occurring.[16]

More recently, Dr. Martin Pall, Professor Emeritus of Biochemistry and Basic Medical Sciences at Washington State University, has built a case that Voltage-Gated Calcium Channel (VGCC) activation in cells from low-intensity EMFs, such as those emitted by cell phones, wireless devices and wireless infrastructure, is a primary mechanism of biological dysfunction. He believes the VGCC activation in cells can explain long-reported association between electromagnetic fields and a wide range of biological changes and health effects, including[17]:

1) Various neuropsychiatric effects, including changes in brain structure and function, changes in various types of psychological responses and changes in behavior.
2) At least eight different endocrine (hormonal) effects.
3) Cardiac effects influencing the electrical control of the heart, including changes in ECGs producing arrhythmias, changes that can be life threatening.
4) Chromosome breaks and other changes in chromosome structure.
5) Histological changes in the testes.
6) Cell death (what is now called apoptosis, a process important in neurodegenerative diseases).
7) Lowered male fertility including lowered sperm quality and function and also lowered female fertility (less studied).
8) Oxidative stress.
9) Changes in calcium fluxes and calcium signaling.
10) Cellular DNA damage including single strand breaks and double strand breaks in cellular DNA and also 8-OHdG in cellular DNA.
11) Cancer which is likely to involve these DNA changes but also increased rates of tumor promotion-like events.
12) Therapeutic effects including stimulation of bone growth.

"We're clearly at a point where we can confidently debunk the industry's argument of more than 20 years that there cannot be a biological mechanism of action from these low-intensity EMFs."

—Martin Pall, PhD
Professor Emeritus in Biochemistry
and Basic Medical Sciences
Washington State University

13) Cataract formation (previously thought to be thermal, now known not to be).

14) Breakdown of the blood-brain barrier.

15) Melatonin depletion and sleep disruption.

Dr. Pall says, "We're clearly at a point where we can confidently debunk the industry's argument of more than 20 years that there cannot be a biological mechanism of action from these low-intensity EMFs. According to industry, the forces electromagnetic fields place on electrically-charged groups in the cell are too weak to produce biological effects. However, the unique structural properties of the VGCC protein can, it turns out, explain why the force on a cell's voltage sensor from low-intensity EMFs are millions of times stronger than are the forces on singly-charged groups elsewhere in the cell.[18] They may be low intensity but with regard to the VGCCs, can have a tremendously powerful impact on the cell. Furthermore, published studies showing that calcium channel blocker drugs block or greatly lower biological effects from electromagnetic fields confirm there is a voltage-gated calcium channel mechanism that is occurring."[19]

While there may be other mechanisms which can lead to biological effects from EMFs, we now know that activation of the VGCC is at least one very important factor that can lead to a range of effects.

Is it not time we start to pay attention, and think more about the 'Wireless Elephant' in the room if we want to get people well and lower health care costs?

After all, we have over half a century of science showing biological effects, while radiation exposures continue to grow ever more pervasive and more powerful.

Are we afraid, I wonder, to recognize this elephant?

"With dramatic increases in reported ASCs (autism spectrum conditions) that are coincident in time with the deployment of wireless technologies, we need aggressive investigation of potential ASC–EMF/RFR links".

—**Martha Herbert, MD**
Assistant Professor of Neurology,
Harvard Medical School; Pediatric
Neurologist and Neuroscientist,
Mass General Hospital; and Author,
*The Autism Revolution: Whole Body
Strategies for Making Life All It Can Be*

Experts are Warning

Indeed, it took decades to have the truth emerge on risks from tobacco, asbestos, and lead paint, but in the case of electromagnetic fields experts warn that, because of the ubiquitous exposures, we must act with urgency to prevent consequences of potentially catastrophic proportions.

Ominously, in 2013, Harvard autism expert, Martha Herbert, MD, published an article indicating that the very same biological changes happening in autism happen with electromagnetic field exposures.[20]

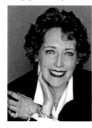 She says the evidence is sufficient now to warrant new public exposure standards, and strong, interim precautionary practices. "With dramatic increases in reported ASCs (autism spectrum conditions) that are coincident in time with the deployment of wireless technologies, we need aggressive investigation of potential ASC–EMF/RFR links", says Dr. Herbert.

Autism now affects approximately 1 in 50 school age children[21], up from 1 in 1,500 in the 1990s, when the widespread proliferation of antenna infrastructure began.[22] MIT Senior Research Scientist Stephanie Seneff of MIT's Computer Science and Artificial Intelligence Laboratory projects 1 in 2 children will be on the autism spectrum by 2032. If there is even a small chance EMFs could be playing a role in the growth of autism, along with other factors, like vaccines, mercury and glyphosate, the topic certainly deserves our immediate attention, given the condition's continued non-stop growth and the seriously alarming projections.

Dr. Herbert says, "EMF/RFR from WiFi and cell towers can exert a disorganizing effect on the ability to learn and remember, and can also be destabilizing to immune and metabolic functions. This will make it harder for some children to learn, particularly those who are already having problems in the first place."

Beyond RF impacts on attention, memory, and behavior, in extreme cases, children are exhibiting signs of "digital dementia", where

"I can say with conviction, in light of the science, and in particular in light of the cellular and DNA science, which has been my focus at Columbia University for several decades, putting radiating antennas in schools (and in close proximity to developing children) is an uninformed choice."

—**Martin Blank, PhD**
Department of Physiology &
Cellular Biophysics
Columbia University

overuse of technology leads to symptoms comparable to dementia in the elderly.[23] We should be aghast that this is occurring to children, and that companies are allowed to push wireless technology on them without regard to the short- or long-term consequences.

In commercial or industrial grade WiFi, found in schools, where the RF radiation is designed to be strong enough to easily go through cement walls, and to handle dozens to hundreds of users, the rate of cardiac arrest in children can be 40x the expected rate. Instead of addressing increasing incidence of heart irregularities in children by turning off the WiFi, some schools are sheepishly addressing the problem by installing defibrillators.[24] This is clearly no solution.

There is a statistically significant increased risk for brain cancer from cell phone use, enough to now upgrade the IARC classification to Group 1 'Carcinogen' from 'Possible Carcinogen' according to recently published studies.[25] Young people who begin using cell phones heavily before age 20 have four to five times more risk of brain cancer by their late 20s.[26] Risk has been shown to increase with years and total hours of use, as would be expected.

David Carpenter, MD, Director of the Institute for Health and the Environment at the University at Albany, a former New York State Department of Health official who ran the state's largest public health laboratory, and who was previously Dean of the School of Public Health at the University at Albany/SUNY, says, "There is clear and strong evidence that intensive use of cell phones increases the risk of brain cancer, tumors of the auditory nerve and cancer of the parotid gland, the salivary gland in the cheek by the ear."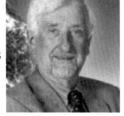

In a letter to a school Board of Trustees, Martin Blank, PhD, of the Department of Physiology and Cellular Biophysics at Columbia University, and author of *"Overpowered: The Dangers of Electromagnetic Radiation (EMF) and What You Can Do About It*," says, "I can say with conviction, in light of the science, and in particular in light of the cellular and DNA science, which has

We are allowing the population to be continually exposed to biologically disturbing wireless technologies that can make people tired, irritable, distracted, depressed, anxious, addicted, unproductive, unfriendly, and feeling like "zombies", and that can also lead to many illnesses, including many serious and life-threatening ones, like brain tumors and other cancers. Significant harm is being done to our society biologically, psychologically, spiritually and economically right before our eyes.

been my focus at Columbia University for several decades, putting radiating antennas in schools (and in close proximity to developing children) is an uninformed choice." He adds, "Assurances that the antennas are within 'FCC guidelines' is meaningless today, given that it is now widely understood that the methodology used to assess exposure levels only accounts for one type of risk from antennas, the thermal effect from the power, not the other known risks, such as non-thermal frequencies, pulsing, signal characteristics, etc. They fail also to consider multiple simultaneous exposures from a variety of sources in the environment, and cumulative exposures over a lifetime. Compliance with FCC guidelines, thus, unfortunately, is not in any way an assurance of safety today, as the guidelines are fundamentally flawed." [27]

In 2015, 190 EMF scientists from 39 countries sent an International EMF Scientist Appeal to the United Nations, saying the World Health Organization has an internal conflicting stance on risks from electromagnetic fields, that needs strengthening, calling for protection of humans and wildlife.[28] Columbia's Dr. Martin Blank was the Appeal's spokesperson. Watch video here:

https://vimeo.com/123468632

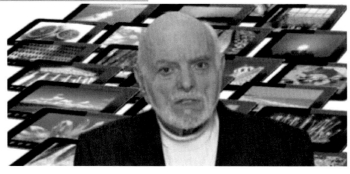

To date, there is evidence of a connection between electromagnetic fields and nine cancers: Glioma (brain cancer), Acoustic Neuroma (tumor on acoustic nerve), Meningioma (tumor of the meninges), Salivary Gland cancer (parotid gland in cheek), Eye Cancer, Testicular Cancer, Leukemia, Thyroid Cancer and Breast Cancer. In five of these cancers, the RF-cancer connection has now been identified in multiple studies and in multiple countries.[29]

To date, there is evidence of a connection between electromagnetic fields and nine cancers: Glioma (brain cancer), Acoustic Neuroma (tumor on acoustic nerve), Meningioma (tumor of the meninges), Salivary Gland cancer (parotid gland in cheek), Eye Cancer, Testicular Cancer, Leukemia, Thyroid Cancer and Breast Cancer.

—L. Lloyd Morgan
Senior Research Fellow
Environmental Health Trust

Approximately 3-5% of people are also estimated to be electrically sensitive in developed countries,[30] with up to 35% mildly electrically sensitive.

Overall, the risks and warnings from scientists the world over do not paint a pretty picture, given that billions of people are now using cell phones and wireless devices, while mistakenly thinking they are safe. Wireless radiation is blanketing employees in offices, the sick in hospitals, travelers in hotels, schoolchildren in schools, people in their homes and bedrooms, and even newborns in the neonatal intensive care unit at one Los Angeles hospital.[31]

Young people of childbearing age have no idea that a fetus' exposure to RF radiation in utero can lead to biological effects, such as effects on the brain and on organs,[32] and to greater instances of emotional and social difficulties later in childhood.[33] Young men don't know that they regularly incur risks to fertility by placing a cell phone in their pants pocket.[34] Elders sleeping near a WiFi router, or near a portable phone, have not been told these exposures can impact cognitive function, or lead to heart irregularities and accelerated aging.[35]

In this video on risks from electromagnetic fields in pregnancy, The Baby Safe Project,[36] a collaboration between Grassroots Environmental Education and Environmental Health Trust, features Yale University's Chair of Obstetrics, Gynecology and Reproductive Sciences and Professor of Molecular, Cellular and Developmental Biology, Dr. Hugh Taylor; Dr. Devra Davis of Environmental Health Trust; and Dr. Leo Trasande from NYU Langone School of Medicine.

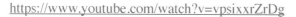
https://www.youtube.com/watch?v=vpsixxrZrDg

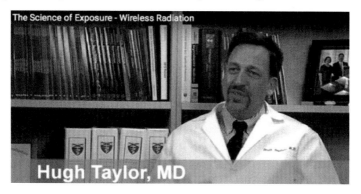

Young people of childbearing age have no idea that a fetus' exposure to RF radiation in utero can lead to biological effects, such as effects on the brain and on organs[32], and to greater instances of emotional and social difficulties later in childhood[33]. Young men don't know they regularly incur risks to fertility by placing a cell phone in their pants pocket.[34] Elders sleeping near a WiFi router, or near a portable phone, have not been told these exposures can impact cognitive function, or lead to heart irregularities and accelerated aging.[35]

People of childbearing age will want to listen carefully to what these experts are saying, and to hear about Dr. Taylor's research in animals showing association between cell phone exposure in utero and symptoms similar to ADHD in offspring.

Devra Davis, PhD says, "Growing evidence tells us that men who want to father healthy babies should follow manufacturers advice and keep phones out of their pockets. Pregnancy is also a time of obvious vulnerability, which is why growing numbers of physicians advise young women to avoid direct exposure to their abdomens of the microwave radiation from cell phones and other wireless transmitting devices." She adds, "People have a fundamental right to know why and how to protect their capacity to have children when and if they choose to do so."

Why is mainstream media ignoring the EMF science when so many people, across all ages, are at risk?

Path of Darkness

Technology developers and manufacturers are also now developing the coming 'Internet of Things'(IoT), where appliances and equipment in our lives will be wirelessly communicating constantly in our homes, but this bodes poorly for health, adding to the present exposures. Why would we want to have wireless radiation from multiple electronics blanketing us in the sanctuary of our home, and without the ability to ever turn them off? Not only is this a health issue, but it is a privacy issue, giving third parties opportunities to study our behaviors in detail, for their commercial purposes.

The FCC has given the green light to move forward with 5th generation (5G) wireless technology, saying it is in the interest of U.S. 'economic activity,' and it recently reallocated parts of the spectrum for it. 5G will utilize ultra-high frequencies (24 to 100+ GHz compared to 2.4 and 5 GHz currently used). Ultra-high frequencies are being permitted, despite research on 2G (GSM) technology showing risks for brain and heart tumors in federal government animal studies; despite 3G (UMTS) technology, though 1000x lower power than 2G, demonstrating several times the cancer risk compared to 2G,[37] ostensibly due to factors other than power, such as modulation (which has been shown to impact

Why would we want to have wireless radiation from multiple electronics blanketing us in the sanctuary of our home, and without the ability to ever turn them off? Not only is this a health issue, but it is a privacy issue, giving third parties opportunities to study our behaviors, in detail, for their commercial purposes.

DNA repair genes[38]); and, despite no health research having yet been conducted on 4G. Nonetheless, outgoing FCC Chairman Tom Wheeler says the country will be covered in a massive deployment of new 5G small cells, on which there has also been no health research. While smaller cells may not be as visible to the public as large cell towers, their presence—and radiation—will be ubiquitous and potentially much more dangerous and biologically disruptive than the radiation we experience today.[39]

It is estimated the 5G market, well underway by developers now, will grow to hundreds of millions of dollars in the next decade.

Of equal concern, large media companies like SpaceX, Google, Facebook, OneWeb, and Outernet are planning to launch WiFi from the air and space, using satellites, balloons and drones. The Google Loon project is an example.[40]

This type of out-of-the-box R&D may give tech employees a sense of purpose, with the novelty being a welcomed stimulant, perhaps, but the real value in connecting all material things in our lives, or in using space for communications, interfering with the atmosphere, when far safer and more energy-efficient hard-wired options exist, has yet to be explained. For our health, of course, we would want to be pushing entirely different 'edges', such as developing meaningful connections among people, and communities, not inanimate machines, and restoring our lost relationship with nature, while using the safer, faster and more secure *wired* technology options that are readily available.

It appears many in technology circles really don't understand this, for they seem to regularly mistake what is only a facsimile of interconnection for our real potential in this regard. There is no intrinsic value in 'integrating us with our information,' or in tethering us to our devices, or in giving data companies the ability to analyze us for their commercial gain, all while using a tremendous amount of energy to sustain wireless equipment and to store data. Product development should instead aim, fundamentally, to meet a *market need*, while being mindful of health, and of environmental and social impacts.

We are in a new business era, and companies will increasingly be called to account for evidence of social responsibility. We are seeing

There is no intrinsic value in 'integrating us with our information,' or in tethering us to our devices, or in giving data companies the ability to analyze us for their commercial gain, while using a tremendous amount of energy to sustain wireless equipment and to store data.

this in the loud demands for non-GMO food, for transparency in product ingredients, in the fair trade movement, in calls for vaccine injury accountability, and, for example, recently in the market response to the first interactive, internet-connected Barbie doll, 'Hello Barbie'. Hello Barbie was lambasted by irate parents over privacy and security concerns, designated "Worst Toy of the Year" by Campaign for Commercial Free Childhood[41] and flopped in the marketplace, achieving only a small fraction of predicted sales.

There are many international groups now calling for wireless companies and their executives to be brought before the International Criminal Court at the Hague for crimes against humanity, as well more and more academics voicing concern about the effects of overuse of technology, and internet addiction, in our culture. And yet ironically, some technology executives who seduce us into thinking non-stop, biologically-disruptive communications technology is actually desirable probably believe that they are doing us a favor. The myopia, and focus on growth at any cost, is profound. As a society, we need to be asking what is at the root of this myopia. How did it happen that so many in technology circles are overlooking one of the most important aspects of life—health—seemingly in denial that we are electromagnetic ourselves? Can it really be only about the greed?

Waking Up—Before the Tipping Point

The day will arrive when the profound injury to our lives and future generations from wireless technologies will be known, including not just the biological and health effects, and links to disease, but the psychological effects, like poorly developed self-worth, and other effects, such as compulsive behaviors, addiction and isolation. We are being conditioned like rats on a treadmill, increasingly addicted to technology and unable to stop taking the drug. Many children have never known the quality of life possible un-tethered to the non-stop universe. They don't know peace, or the sense of safety and inner guidance possible in complete stillness, when one is deeply connected to the natural world, or in community, and not connected to man-made electronics.

What we are increasingly sacrificing in the modern wireless world are relationships of meaning and fulfillment among people, and the awareness that humans and the ecosystem are intended to live in an

The myopia, and focus on growth at any cost, is profound. As a society we need to be asking what is at the root of this myopia. How did it happen that so many in technology circles are overlooking one of the most important aspects of life—health— seemingly in denial that we are electromagnetic ourselves?

active, living, supportive and joyful relationship. Instead, many people, including children, are attached to the stimulant of technology, 'eating the apple' so to speak, ignoring the Garden of Eden before us. We are on a path of decay and decline, and will remain on this path as long as we are still captured by, and addicted to, the stimuli.

A day of reckoning will arrive. Like with young children without impulse control, individuals, adults and children alike, will have to learn their own lessons on this the hard way, seeing the most important things evaporate, beginning with relationships and support systems. This is already happening across all age groups. For all of the 'interconnectedness' promised by technology, people appear less connected in the true sense of the word, and lonelier than ever.

And it is not just humans who are hurting from exposures to radiation. In 2014, the U.S. Department of the Interior said that the FCC standards for radiofrequency radiation do not adequately protect wildlife. This was a watershed moment. I continue to wonder when public sector leaders in this country will not only acknowledge the impact of this radiation on humans, animals, plants and the ecosystem (in droves), but act on it with urgency. What do people have their minds on that could be more important than a foreboding human health and environmental catastrophe from electromagnetic fields that will ultimately impact our sustainability? Indeed, we need a complete rethinking of the way we live on this Earth, in so many regards.

It is important to understand that the evidence for biological effects from this radiation is not new. Evidence of harm dates back decades to military research, decades before there even was a consumer cell phone or wireless industry. It may not have mattered so much in the early years of these technologies, when users were in military settings, and the exposures were not at all widespread. But today, we are living in a dense sea of radiation, day and night. And exposures are accelerating at a rapid pace, and will continue to get worse unless people, including policymakers, unite to question what is happening in our living environment.

The list of known biological effects is now very long, and presents a compelling rationale for rapidly scrapping the way the FCC assesses cell phone and wireless safety, and for developing exposure guidelines

The day will arrive when the profound injury to our lives and future generations from wireless technologies will be known, including not just the biological and health effects, and links to disease, but the psychological effects, like poorly developed self-worth, and other effects, such as compulsive behaviors, addiction and isolation.

that consider not only any thermal effects of the radiation, but the non-thermal (non-heating), and other effects, as well. Martin Blank, PhD and Reeba Goodman, PhD of Columbia University have wisely suggested using changes in DNA biochemistry as a definitive measure of risk across all the different types of frequencies.[42]

Given that we have FCC regulators with links to the wireless industry and significant conflicts of interest, prospects for voluntary change at the FCC are slim. It will likely be the legal system that will ultimately drive change.

A case under the Americans with Disabilities Act is underway in Massachusetts by parents of a 12-year-old experiencing electrosensitivity symptoms from 5Ghz WiFi at a private school, seeking accommodation for the child. Expert hearings are expected to be completed shortly, and a judicial decision will be made on whether the science is substantial enough to support the condition 'electrosensitivity'. The lawsuit would then proceed to either a judicial decision or a jury trial.

In a multi-party lawsuit on cell phone risks (Murray et al v. Motorola et al) in 2014, Judge Frederick H. Weisberg, said:

"If there is even a reasonable possibility that cell phone radiation is carcinogenic, the time for action in the public health and regulatory sectors is upon us. Even though the financial and social cost of restricting such devices would be significant, those costs pale in comparison to the cost in human lives from doing nothing, only to discover thirty or forty years from now that the early signs were pointing in the right direction. If the probability of carcinogenicity is low, but the magnitude of the potential harm is high, good public policy dictates that the risk should not be ignored."

But we cannot afford to wait for government, the legal system, or the health care system to effectively respond before acting to protect and preserve our biology. People can do a lot now preventatively to protect health, if they understand the risks, while also encouraging an appropriate response from our government, especially Congress.
See **50+ EMF Safety Tips and Insights** (http://tinyurl.com/nmbyqhs) and **For Parents to Know** (http://tinyurl.com/hedbvxl).

In a multi-party lawsuit on cell phone risks (*Murray et al v. Motorola et al*) in 2014, Judge Frederick H. Weisberg, said:

"If there is even a reasonable possibility that cell phone radiation is carcinogenic, the time for action in the public health and regulatory sectors is upon us. Even though the financial and social cost of restricting such devices would be significant, those costs pale in comparison to the cost in human lives from doing nothing, only to discover thirty or forty years from now that the early signs were pointing in the right direction. If the probability of carcinogenicity is low, but the magnitude of the potential harm is high, good public policy dictates that the risk should not be ignored."

Connection to Costs

So let's turn back to prevention, and our health care system. Presently, we are paying for a bloated, expensive, pharmaceutical and treatment-oriented health care system that is not educating people about the need to minimize exposures to wireless radiation (or other environmental factors) when a lot of peoples' problems stem from these exposures. Instead, we wait until the symptoms appear and then treat them with pharmaceuticals, modulating physiology, but never addressing the roots of the problem. This is a no-win situation.

People are given sleeping pills, for example, instead of being told to try turning off the wireless router, or heart medications, instead of being told wireless radiation can lead to heart irregularities (in one study increasing the heart rate in 40% of subjects—almost doubling the rate in one subject)[43]. Children by the millions are being given ADHD medications, while increasingly tethered to biologically disturbing wireless devices that could be contributing to attention difficulties. Homeowners across the country do not know the new radiating utility meters are making them sick, or that they can, in many cases, opt-out.[44] The list goes on. Our health is being eroded by these exposures, yet many are under our daily control.

In a Harvard Safra Center for Ethics report, *"Captured Agency: How the Federal Communications Commission is Dominated by the Industries it Presumably Regulates,"* the authors said 'public ignorance' is the best ally of industry. But this ignorance about wireless impacts won't last. People are increasingly motivated to find solutions to their health challenges themselves, in part due to the new, very high deductible insurance plans. This is good. As health costs rise higher and higher, sooner or later more and more people will likely connect the dots between a wide range of health challenges and wireless devices and infrastructure—ranging from inflammation-related problems, like joint pain, to neurological diseases, heart irregularities, brain tumors, low fertility, and cancers—and decide to minimize their personal exposures.

Captured Agency:
How the Federal Communications Commission Is Dominated by the Industries It Presumably Regulates

Significant harm is being done to our society biologically, psychologically, spiritually and economically right before our eyes.

While the new health insurance mandate aims to assure the health care system can be there for people's health care costs, such as expensive (and for most people, prohibitive) hospitalization costs, capping patients annual out-of-pocket costs, the system certainly isn't serving patients' interests in prevention now, or attempting to understand the root sources of imbalance driving the growth in chronic illnesses in the first place, such as electromagnetic fields. It's worthwhile to attempt to make care affordable for people, but the current approach is trying to patch the health care system way downstream, well after many, if not most, illnesses could have been prevented.

Only when we start focusing on *root sources* of imbalances, like EMFs, as well as food and water toxicity, chemicals in every day products, GMOs, glyphosate, pharmaceuticals, vaccines, poor nutrition, etc., and decide to teach people how to live healthily, will we be offering the quality of care that has a chance of actually getting people better. Otherwise, without telling people the truth on these matters, we've essentially given up on peoples' health potential from the get-go.

When it comes to EMFs, we are allowing the population to be continually exposed to biologically disturbing wireless technologies that can make people tired, irritable, distracted, depressed, anxious, addicted, unproductive, unfriendly, and feeling like 'zombies', and that can lead to many illnesses, including many serious and life-threatening ones, like brain tumors. Significant harm is being done to our society biologically, psychologically, spiritually and economically right before our eyes. A poll by Common Sense Media reported on by CNN recently indicated half of teenagers believe they are addicted to their smart phones.[45]

Isn't it time we courageously acknowledge the damaging impact of cell phones and wireless technologies, and find a new path forward?

Why should we, in essence, be agreeing to be the collateral damage of the wireless industry's misguided values that are damaging humans, animals and nature, and especially children, on an unprecedented scale, for their commercial gain?

I encourage all to stand up for health, start asking questions and demand that this dark industry, that is propagating illness and death, be properly regulated to protect our health and that of future generations.

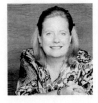

The Author: Camilla Rees, MBA is an internationally respected researcher and educator on the biological and health effects of electromagnetic fields, and co-author of *"Public Health SOS: The Shadow Side of the Wireless Revolution"*. She founded ElectromagneticHealth.org (www.ElectromagneticHealth.org) and Campaign for Radiation Free Schools (Facebook), and co-founded the International EMF Alliance. Camilla is a Senior Policy Advisor to the National Institute for Science, Law and Public Policy; Advisory Board member of the International Institute for Building-Biology™ & Ecology; a Voting Member of the U.S. Health Freedom Congress; and EMF Advisor to Citizens for Health, Radiation Research Trust (U.K.) and Mercola.com.

References

1. Partnership to Fight Chronic Disease report http://www.fightchronicdisease.org/sites/default/files/docs/GrowingCrisisofChronicDiseaseintheUSfactsheet_81009.pdf
2. Scientific American, May 27, 2016. http://www.scientificamerican.com/article/major-cell-phone-radiation-study-reignites-cancer-questions/
3. BioInitiative and Ecolog Reports. Thousands of studies showing biological effects from low intensity radiation were synthesized in the BioInitiative Report (last update 2012, 2014) (www.BioInitiative.org). Many other reviews of the science exist, such as the Ecolog Report, a review commissioned by T-Mobile and Deutsche Telecom MobilNet GmbH, prepared in 2000, which outlined much of the science showing biological effects from cell phone radiation, including gene toxicity, impacts on cellular processes, effects on the immune system, central nervous system, hormone systems and connections with cancer and infertility (http://bemri.org/hese-uk/en/niemr/ecologsumd240.html?content_type=&style=print).
4. WHO/IARC Classified Radiofrequency Electromagnetic Fields as Possibly Carcinogenic to Humans, http://electromagnetichealth.org/electromagnetic-health-blog/iarc-rf-carc/
5. Map of global WiFi Networks from Space. http://www.businessinsider.com/wi-fi-map-of-largest-cities-in-the-world-2015-9
6. Information Week http://www.informationweek.com/mobile/mobile-devices/gartner-21-billion-iot-devices-to-invade-by-2020/d/d-id/1323081
7. Minnesota Geriatrics http://www.minnesotageriatrics.org/Topics_october_15.pdf; American Society of Consulting Pharmacists
8. Emails Dr. Henry Lai, University of Washington, April 11-17. 2016
9. BioInitiative Report www.BioInitiative.org
10. Victoria Dunckley, MD at Commonwealth Club of California https://vimeo.com/132159417
11. Letter to Parents on Fertility and Other Risks to Children from Wireless Technologies http://electromagnetichealth.org/electromagnetic-health-blog/letter-to-parents/
12. BioInitiative Report, www.BioInitiative.org
13. Electrosensitivity U.K., http://www.es-uk.info/
14. Ecolog Report commissioned by T-Mobile and Deutsche Telecom, http://electromagnetichealth.org/electromagnetic-health-blog/t-mobile-deutsche/
15. ICEMS Report, http://electromagnetichealth.org/electromagnetic-health-blog/icems
16. Kirschvink JL: Bioelectromagnetics 17(3):187-194, 1996
17. Email received from Dr. Martin Pall 4/13/16
18. Rev Environ Health. 2015;30(2):99-116. doi: 10.1515/reveh-2015-0001. http://www.ncbi.nlm.nih.gov/pubmed/25879308
19. J Cell Mol Med. 2013 Aug; 17(8): 958–965. http://www.ncbi.nlm.nih.gov/pmc/articles/PMC3780531/
20. Harvard Autism Researcher Warns. http://www.marthaherbert.org/library/Herbert-Sage-2013-Autism-EMF-PlausibilityPathophysiologicalLink-Part21.pdf
21. Reuters http://www.reuters.com/article/us-usa-autism-idUSBRE92J0YX20130320
22. NIMH. http://www.nimh.nih.gov/about/director/2009/nimhs-response-to-new-hrsa-autism-prevalence-estimate.shtml

23. Digital Dementia. https://vimeo.com/71749330; http://www.alzheimers.net/2013-11-12/overuse-of-technology-can-lead-to-digital-dementia/
24. Safety Code 6 testimony by Rodney Palmer to the Royal Society of Canada, https://www.youtube.com/watch?v=uSBwyrZOGQ0
25. Lennart Hardell, MD. https://lennarthardellenglish.wordpress.com/category/iarc/
26. Hardell & Carlberg, Mobile phones, cordless phones and the risk for brain tumours. International Journal of Oncology 35: 5-17, 2009
27. Martin Blank, PhD Letter http://electromagnetichealth.org/wp-content/uploads/2016/01/blank.pdf
28. EMF Scientist Appeal to UN. https://emfscientist.org/
29. L. Lloyd Morgan, Senior Research Fellow, Environmental Health Trust
30. Reported functional impairments of electrohypersensitive Japanese: A questionnaire survey http://www.sciencedirect.com/science/article/pii/S0928468012000442
31. Cedars Sinai, Los Angeles, iPads in Neonatal Intensive Care. https://www.cedars-sinai.edu/About-Us/HH-Landing-Pages/iPads-Help-New-Moms-Connect-With-Their-Infants-in-the-Neonatal-Intensive-Care-Unit.aspx
32. Commonwealth Club of California, June 22, 2015. Dr. Nesrin Seyhan, https://vimeo.com/132881352, and Suleyman Kaplan, MD, https://vimeo.com/132987053
33. UCLA & Danish study-Social-Emotional Effects Later in Life from Fetal Exposure, http://ph.ucla.edu/news/press-release/2011/mar/study-questions-safety-childrens-exposure-cell-phones-during-prenatal
34. Letter to Parents on Fertility and Other Risks to Children from Wireless Technologies by Camilla Rees of ElectromagneticHealth.org, http://electromagnetichealth.org/electromagnetic-health-blog/letter-to-parents/
35. Rapid Aging Syndrome video by Magda Havas, PhD, https://www.youtube.com/watch?v=6z9Dpe66SzE&feature=player_embedded#at=14
36. The BabySafe Project, http://www.babysafeproject.org/the-science/
37. Mercola.com, http://articles.mercola.com/sites/articles/archive/2015/01/06/cell-phone-use-brain-cancer-risk.aspx ; International Journal of Oncology http://www.ncbi.nlm.nih.gov/pmc/articles/PMC3829779/
38. IY Belyaev, Impairment of DNA Repair Genes. https://www.youtube.com/watch?v=yCHlhmX9Bio
39. LA Times on 5G. http://www.latimes.com/business/la-fi-cellphone-5g-health-20160808-snap-story.html
40. C4ST, http://c4st.org/international-coalition-objects-to-googles-project-loon/
41. Fortune, Hello Barbie, http://fortune.com/2015/12/08/worst-toy-year/
42. Electromagnetic Biology and Medicine, June 7, 2012, Electromagnetic fields and health: DNA-based dosimetry http://www.tandfonline.com/doi/abs/10.3109/15368378.2011.624662
43. Radiation from Cordless Phones Cause Heart Irregularities. http://electromagnetichealth.org/electromagnetic-health-blog/cordless-heart/
44. Smart Meters—not so Smart - How Dangerous and Expensive Became "Smart" - An Exposé of the "Smart Grid", Amy Worthington http://www.westonaprice.org/health-topics/smart-meters-not-so-smart/
45. Half of Teenagers Addicted to Smart Phones http://www.cnn.com/2016/05/03/health/teens-cell-phone-addiction-parents/

Additional Resources

Documentaries

 Public Exposure: DNA, Democracy and the Wireless Revolution (2001)

 Full Signal: The Hidden Cost of Cell Phones (2011)

 Resonance: Beings of Frequency (2013)

 Take Back Your Power (2013)

 Mobilize (2014, 2016)

 Screenagers (2016)

EMF Exposure Assessment

International Institute for Building Biology™ and Ecology trains environmental consultants in home assessment and remediation, including regarding exposures to multiple types of electromagnetic fields. Consultants have varying levels of experience. See directory at www.hbelc.org

Industrial hygienists work in corporate and industrial settings, and have different degrees of experience in EMF assessment and remediation. See American Industrial Hygiene Association. www.aiha.org

Many activists and health educators have developed competence in EMF assessment and remediation, and may be all one needs to make impactful changes to support health, though they may have no formal training or technical degree. See health advocacy groups associated with the International EMF Alliance at www.iemfa.org to find local groups who may be able to help you. To buy a meter, and for other assessment and remediation supplies, go to www.EMFSafetyStore.com

National Institute for Science, Law & Public Policy

The National Institute for Science, Law & Public Policy (NISLAPP) was founded in 1978 to bridge the gap between scientific uncertainties and the need for laws protecting public health and safety. Its overriding objective is to bring practitioners of science and law together to develop intelligent policy that best serves all interested parties in a given controversy. Its focus is on the points at which these two disciplines converge.

Supporting Our Work

Thank you for taking the time to read *The Wireless Elephant in the Room*. Would you be able to help us to print and widely distribute this booklet, such as to government officials, schools, health practitioners, churches and journalists?

We thank you wholeheartedly for any assistance you can offer. It is only through citizens at the grassroots becoming educated that we will be able to make progress at the federal level, where critical changes to protect human health, animals and nature must take place. We are grateful for whatever you can give.

Please send contributions to the 501(c)(3) non-profit National Institute for Science, Law & Public Policy at 1601 18th Street, NW, Suite 4, Washington, DC 20009. Earmark your donation for the 'EMF Education Project'. Or, consider donating online via: http://manhattanneighbors.org/we-donate/

If you would consider making a major gift or bequest, please contact Camilla Rees at 415-992-5093 or Camilla@ManhattanNeighbors.org.

Thank you very much for your support.

Made in the USA
Columbia, SC
02 January 2019